Of
Potions

Of Potions

A beginner's text book

A basic understanding of how the magic of nature can be used to maintain health of spirit and soul. Basic measures are provided to start with. Recognize plant's energy by taste. Choose the right potion to suite the need. Answers to questions asked in the beginning of the journey.

This book is not intended as a medical reference or as a guide for herbalist. The author is not a physician or an herbalist. The illustrations in this book are not intended for identification. The intent of this book is to spark an interest in exploring the power held within the natural surroundings of our world. The application of information in this book is at the readers own discretion and risk.

ISBN 978-0-9825793-6-7

Jeff Cross

Published by JCrossBooks.com
Knowledge and Entertainment

In Acknowledgement

I would like to express a special thanks to Valarie January for her help and insight.

I would like to express our appreciation to Wikimedia Commons for making public domain artwork available.

Of Potions

Beginners Textbook

The art of potion making is of the light and of the dark and the potion maker must find a balance between the two. As in all things, as in any craft, as in life itself, knowledge must be acquired from accurate information. The making of potions is a practiced art and it must be treated as such. One must document with great accuracy all one does and refer to actions and doses to enhance the outcome of works. The following measures are a foundation. Build on this foundation and change it as the need be to obtain the balance required.

Treat each person as the individual they are. Treat each herb with the respect it deserves as the magic within has powers that reach much more than what may be expected. One herb can affect up to sixteen organs. When one mixes several herbs to accommodate a specific reaction, the reaction may have side effects that are unexpected.

Many of the common strengths that herbs have can be tasted or otherwise recognized by the tongue or nose. It is important one learns to recognize these tastes as they are the similar everywhere. In this way one is able to make potions where ever they go even though one is not familiar with the local flora.

Many potion makers learn to mix potions from many different materials to create very specialized results. As one beginning the craft, one should learn each herb separately. One plant has magic that spans across many organs and has powers that affect a person in many different ways. This information must be studied separately and recorded accurately. If one mixes materials together, and each material has a unique action on the benefactor, one knows not what each material is responsible for.

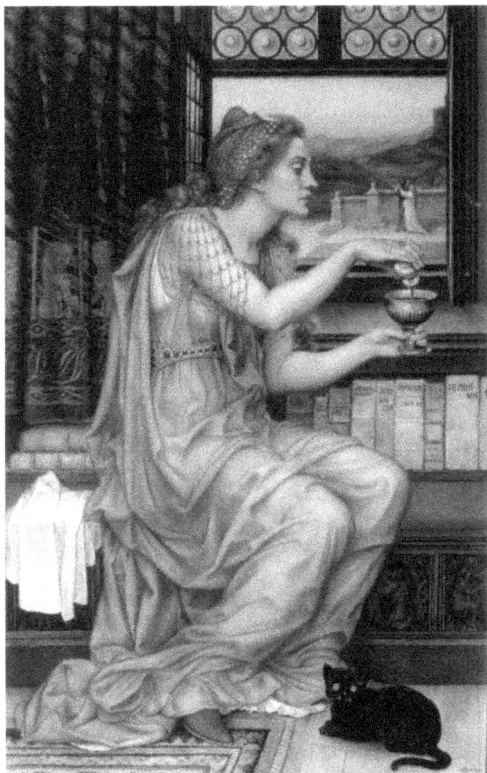

One

Seven Basic Potion Making Methods and Other Applications

An *Infusion* is the first method of potion making. Place the herb into an open vessel may it be crushed or whole, it should lay in the lower portion of the container. Pour upon it pure water that has been heated to boil. Cover the material completely and allow it to steep for up to a half of an hour. Pour off the tea withholding the solids. Infusions may be consumed as a tea or applied topically.

A *Decoction* is the second method of bringing the power of an herb out to a useful and measurable potion. Using pure water place sixteen parts water to one part herb and bring to a slow boil. Set off fire and steep for up to one half hour. Some softer herbs may require as little as eight parts water to one part herb. Pour off the decoction withholding the solid parts. When preparing a fresh plant with roots, stem and leaves, place the roots into the vessel first. The color of the decoction must be memorized as this determines its strength. Decoctions may be consumed as a tea or applied topically.

A *Tincture* is the third of the three most common potion formulas. One part herb resting covered in two parts of alcohol in a tightly closed vessel within a dark cupboard for a period of not less than fourteen days. The plant material may be fresh or dried. Depending on the tincture, the mixture may be agitated once or twice a day during this period. When the material is ready, the liquid is strained off and used or further processed with a low heat to evaporate the alcohol making the tincture stronger. Tinctures may be added to food, drink or intermingled with other potions. Tinctures may also be applied topically. A tincture will render forty times the magic that an infusion will make. Do not use with children.

Oil Infusions are made by placing the herb in a cheese cloth and steeping it in warmed oil. A ratio of one to sixteen should be used and the oil must be of a light variety such as virgin olive or almond. Continue heating the infusion until the plant has lost its color or the oil has the fragrance of the herb. This method is required on root and bark as a tincture lacks the power to withdraw the magic. The infusion is applied topically as soon as it has cooled.

An *Oil Tincture* would use the same ration of oil and herb as an infusion, but the tincture would not be heated. The material must be placed in the cupboard for a minimum of fourteen days and usually for a full cycle of the moon. The oil is used without removing the herbs within and is applied topically.

Honey Infusions use the healing power of the honey to accentuate the power of an herb or herb mixture. Honey is one of the most powerful natural victual in existence. Honey does not spoil, it is a natural antibiotic and it will absorb the useful elements from herbs. Warm the honey by placing the vessel into a second vessel of water. Heat to thin but do not boil the honey. Place the herb into the honey and store for twenty eight days within a cupboard. Remove and warm as before to thin the honey. Drain the herbs out and use the honey topically or internally.

A *Balm* is a potion mixed into a heavy oil, honey, whipped wax or lard. One may use an herb, tincture or an infusion with one of the substrates mentioned before to keep the herbs power in contact with the skin without cover or protection such as a bandage. When using a water based decoction or infusion, it is difficult to keep the oils or lard from separating from the balm's base material. Never use petroleum products as a substitute.

A *Wash* is a mild infusion made for topical application only. Use one part herb in thirty parts pure boiling water. Steep until potion is warm to the touch and apply to afflicted area.

A *Poultice* is a thick paste made of crushed herb and moistened with water or oil. It is normally warmed and applied to a bandage and placed on the affected part of the body. In some cases the dregs of an infusion or decoction is used as a poultice.

Two

Tools of the Practice

Vessels must be of a glass that can be heated to boil oils. Utensils for cutting and small measures must be of silver or a metal that will not allow leaching. Vessels for storage must be of glass of green or of amber or of a color to prevent light from diminishing the strength of its contents. Liquids must never be stored in glass of blue, though powders may.

Tools of measure must be of the highest of quality attainable. The gathering of herbs must be weighed before and after they are dried. They must be weighed after they are processed into crushed particles or after they are cut into pieces.

Liquids must be accurately measured and documented so that the prescribed amount will be exact. Therefore, measuring vessels must remain marked and clean. Utensils must be maintained in a usable and accurate manner. Cutting tools must be kept sharp.

Two mortar and pestle must be at hand, one of stone for seeds, nuts and dried roots. The other of Holly wood for leafs, fresh seeds, blooms, stems and softer materials.

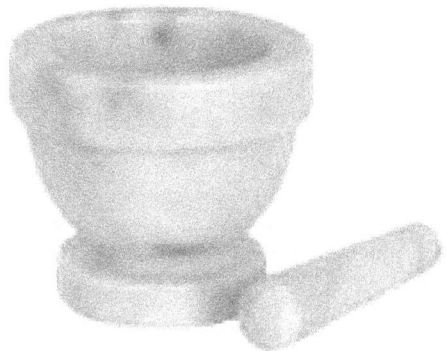

A cupboard must be large enough to store completed potions as well as potions being made. Most tinctures will no longer be of quality to use after a year and some essential oils will only last for two years. Balms may not last a month without being kept cool. Infusions and decoctions will only last a few days. One will need to dry and store herbs through the winter and collect them again when they are ready. A dark, cool and dry place to store dried plant material must be at hand.

Parchment and pen must be on hand to document all actions and reactions, recipes and concoctions. It is best to document all actions with dates. This will assist in reproducing the potion with more accuracy.

Fine cutting shears are to be used in harvesting, for the breaking off of limbs must not be permitted. A small saw may be required at times to remove a branch to obtain the bark.

A magnifying glass of 20X may be required to identify some of the plants collected. A difference of texture of stems can mean the difference between life and death. Research and obtain the clearest texts to carry for identification. Identification is not covered within this text as this book is for the beginner.

Three

Material of Substrate and of Dilution

The most common solvent used is **Water**. The source of water must be confirmed pure and any water stored must not be allowed to sit for more than seven days. Fresh pure water must be stored in clean glass containers in a well lit place, for the sun purifies and the moon blesses. *Water is used to dissolve or extract from herbs, sugars, alkaloids, gums, tannins, pectin, bitter compounds, and starch.*

For the making of tinctures, a solvent must be used. **Alcohol** is the most common type of solvent and it too must be of the highest of quality. When purchasing alcohol, search for a clear drink that is of one hundred-proof. One hundred-proof is fifty percent alcohol and fifty percent water. The best results come from the use of forty-five to fifty percent alcohol. *This type of solvent would be used to extract salts, sugars, alkaloids, tannins and enzymes.*

Oil of plants such as olives or safflower must be of the purest available. Stay away from oils of the beast as this material is detrimental to the recipient and is of the darkness as well. Through infusion or tincture, the magic of an herb will migrate into the oil. Oil is essential in preventing quick evaporation when applying topically.

Vinegar is used in the preparation of some infusions, decoctions and tinctures. Not only does the vinegar have value in itself, *but it helps to bring forth sugars, glycosides and tannins.* To make a tincture with vinegar, use an herb to vinegar ration of one to five and allow the tincture to set in the cupboard for one half the phase of the moon. Agitate it daily. Normally the best vinegar to use is apple cider vinegar. Apple cider vinegar has medicinal qualities of its own. Be cautious with any vinegar as it can burn ones skin. If taking it orally, it must be diluted.

Bees Wax should be collected and stored in a cool place. Melt the wax down and remove all unclean portions. Pour into pads of a measured amount and cool. Bees wax melts at a temperature just above the normal body temperature. It is the perfect substrate for creating a balm. Use oil tincture to mix with wax or mix a decoction with a small amount of olive oil and heat until the water evaporates completely and then add bees wax. This balm must simmer at 150 degrees Fahrenheit until one is pleased with the consistency. Use a balm for beauty products or minor skin ailments.

Four

Wildcrafting

The collection of plant material for the use of potions and food is also known as wildcrafting. One must use wisdom in collecting from the mother. Greed must not prevail. Give back more than you take. Give thanks in action and in spirit, for Karma walks with Mother.

To know when to collect a particular plant, one must know what part of the plant one intends to use. The common parts are the root, inner bark of the root, leaves, blooms, stems, bark and sap.

The roots are collected in the fall when the plants energy moves down. The best time is after the equinox on the new moon.

Leaves are collected in the spring before the plant flowers. Leaves and flowers are best collected on the full moon.

Collect flowers as they have just bloomed, as this is when the most magic resides within them. A few potions may require buds.

The bark would best be collected in the spring or the fall whilst the moon is three-quarter waning. Never remove bark from a standing tree. This opens a wound that will allow sickness or pests to enter.

Seeds are at their peak just before they fall. The birds will tell you when they are ready.

Saps are harvested in the fall or the spring as it is in transit at this time.

When collecting leaves in the day, choose the morning time after the dew is gone, yet before the heat has set in. Harvesting roots should occur in the warmer part of the day on into the evening before the cold sets in.

Plants should be used fresh if possible. To maintain a good stock for any length of time, one must carefully dry the plants. Whole plants are hung from the bottom and allowed to air dry in the darkness. Damp roots or damp leaves are cut into thin slices and laid on a screen or strung on threads in darkness with dry air moving around them.

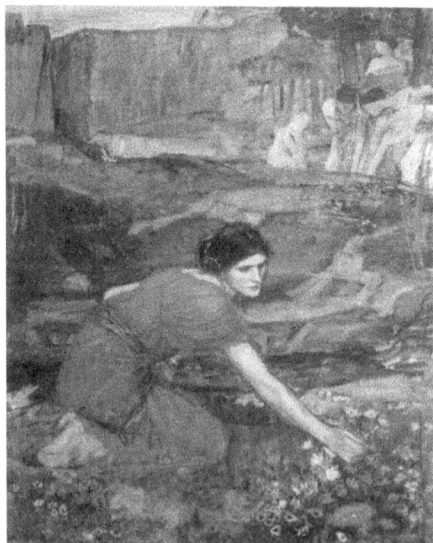

Seeds may be collected from blooms by drying the blooms in the upright position and turning them over a vessel after drying.

Avoid wildcrafting along heavy traveled roadways, near industries, or other places where traffic or chemicals may contaminate the fauna.

Five

Terms One Should Know

Analgesic – A pain killer

Antacid – Neutralizes acid in the stomach

Antibiotic –Kills or slows the reproduction of bacteria

Antihistamine – Slows or stops the production of histamine

Anti-inflammatory – Prevent or reduces inflammation. Not the same as an astringent

Antifungal – Kills or slows the reproduction of fungi

Antimicrobial – Kills or slows the reproduction of microorganisms such as fungi, bacteria or protozoan

Antipruritic – Stops or eases an itch

Antipyretic – Reduces fever, same as febrifuge

Antiseptic – Kills germs and reduces chances of infection

Aphrodisiac – Corrects impotence by increasing sexual desire

Aromatics – An herb that stimulates gastrointestinal mucus membranes by means of odor, aiding in digestion

Astringent – A material that tends to shrink tissue

Antispasmodic – A material that suppresses muscle spasms

Bile – A fluid of the liver that the body uses to emulsify fats in the small intestines

Cathartic – An herb that quickly evacuates the upper intestines and bowels by promoting the flow of bile

Demulcent – Is soothing to inflamed tissue and is commonly used for mucus membranes

Diuretic –Increases the urine and helps remove body fluid

Deobstruent – An herb used to open or clear the fluid ducts and secretions of the body

Discutient – Dissolve tumors or abnormal growths by topical application

Emetic – Induces vomiting

Expectorant – A material that helps to eliminate mucus from the upper respiratory tract

Febrifuge – Reduces fever, same as antipyretic

Fomentation – Applying moist heat to ease local pain by increasing the flow of blood to the affected area

Laxative – Soften stool, usually in the colon, to allow easier evacuation of the bowel

Hemostatic – Stops bleeding by contracting the blood vessels or tissue. Opposite of Hemorrhagic

Hepatic – Affecting the liver or its function

Lithotriptic – Herbs help to dissolve gall stones and gravel

Mucilage – Thick gummy substance obtained from plants that have soothing properties when applied topically

Nervine – Acts upon the nerves in a sedative manor

Pectoral – Herbs that pertain to the chest or lungs

Sedative – Induces sedation, sleep or relaxes

Sialagogue – Stimulates the flow of saliva from the salivary glands

Stimulant – Increases mental activity or metabolism

Styptic – Stops bleeding by contracting the blood vessels or tissue. Similar to astringent, like Hemostatic

Vulnerary – A remedy that promotes healing or has curative powers.

Six

Benefactor

Each person you deal with is unique. Each person is also alike in many ways. The statement sounds conflictive, and it is not easy to practice. One must remember the balance in life. As one needs light they also need dark. As one needs water one also needs to be dry. One needs warmth yet one needs to be cooled. This applies to the soul and to the spirit. One needs to feel good as they also need to feel good about themselves.

When a person is hot and damp, one must give them a cool dry place. This will sway the person back into balance. If a person feels cloudy; a sunny feeling must be applied to counter the imbalance. A person that is out of balance will display one or more of the characteristics on the next page. It is important to observe the person and speak to them so one understands which characteristics the person has and why. The goal is to find the root cause.

In most cases a combination of several characteristics will be present. As all herbs and potions treat more than one complication, one must be careful to prevent throwing another organ out of balance while treating the other. Take notice which imbalances are of the body and which ones are of the spirit. They are equally important and may need to be treated separately or together.

Characteristics that are darker and affect the physical body are:

Cold	Fixed
Wet	Dull
Heavy	Soft
Coarse	Smooth
Solid	Cloudy

Characteristics that are opposite to those above are of the light and affect ones energy and vitality:

Hot	Mobile
Dry	Sharp
Light	Hard
Fine	Rough
Fluid	Sunny

The darker characteristics are cooling and the lighter ones are warming by nature.

Each characteristic has an opposite. Therefore light balances dark and dark balances light. By understanding the person, one will understand how to treat the imbalance. When a person demonstrates they have heavy and dull qualities, then one focuses on a potion that increases light and sharp characteristics. The characteristics of potions may either react or contain the same characteristics that are described above. One must search for an ingredient that reflects the curative nature, or the result desired. In simplistic terms, when one is hot and tired they desire a meal that cools and refreshes. The same simple evaluation of a potion must be sought yet being careful to maintain balance in other areas.

While using plants that are in their whole state, an unbalanced reaction is not likely to occur. Before a plant is altered by man's hand, it is already in balance.

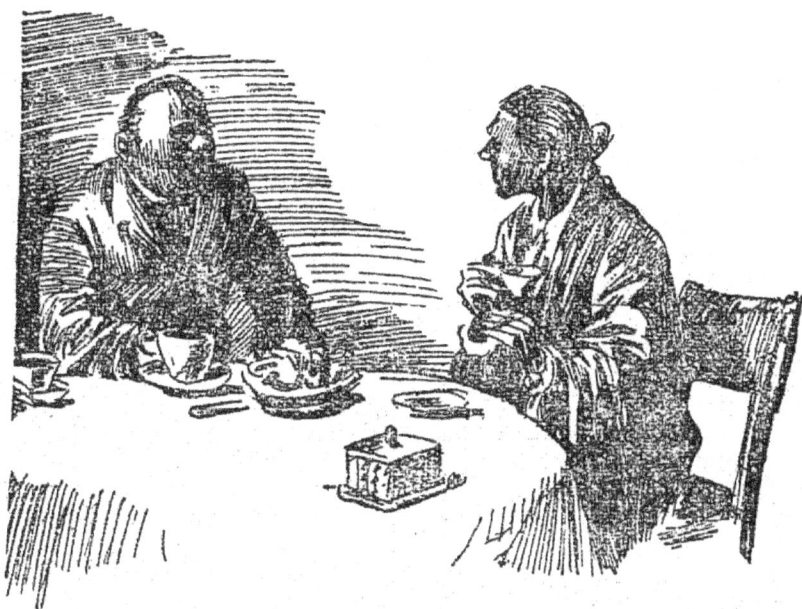

Seven

Taste of Herbs

There are five tastes of herbs that define their magic. Most herbs will have a combination of more than one taste or texture. Each taste can be attached to a general reaction. But the different combinations of taste and texture will cause a unique action in itself. The secondary tastes can be considered less than significant if it will not push another system out of balance.

Sour - Herbs with a sour taste are cooling to organs and tissues. Some have sedative qualities. When the benefactor you are caring for is hot, these herbs are cooling. When the benefactor is excited, these herbs are settling. The magic protects or maintains.

Pungent - Herbs that are hot on the tongue and lips are warming and stimulate cold tissues. They are also antiseptic. Many are an antihistamine. They work on the lungs and sinus. The magic pushes up and out.

Salty - Herbs that are salty tend to moisten tissues and reduce loss of moisture. They have many minerals. If a benefactor is suffering from loss of water such as diarrhea, a salty tasting herb would be considered. They affect the kidneys and detoxify. The magic slows.

Bitter - Herbs that have a bitter taste remove the dampness and aid in increasing out go. Some are laxative. Most bitter

17

tasting herbs affect the digestive tract and detoxify. The magic will push downward and out.

Sweet - Herbs with a sweet taste increases moisture by increasing carbohydrates. They will work on the digestive tract and lower cleansing organs. The magic is sticky and will tend to hold fast.

*Astringen*t - Herbs that are puckering and draw out moisture tend to tighten tissues and create a tension in the organs. These are helpful in reducing bleeding in open wounds. The magic draws inward.

Herbs that are **sharp** tend to relax the tissues and muscles. They are also antispasmodic.

Herbs that are *fragrant* are drying and push up and out.

Cold herbs will cause one to contract and is usually sweet as well.

An herb that is **hot** in nature can quickly warm a person from inside and caution must be taken to prevent overheating.

Eight

Of Blood

Thin Blood flows very freely through the body. People that have naturally thin blood will normally have long thin bones. One may have trouble keeping warm. This condition may weaken the kidneys. A person will feel weak or exhausted especially after perspiring, urinating or having diarrhea. The skin will feel damp and cold. The person may have lines running down the sides of their tongue. An astringent must be provided to tighten up the organs to prevent the loss of water. White oak bark or blueberry leaf may be considered.

When the blood is oily it is said to be **thick blood**. People that have thick blood in their heritage will normally have large thick bones. Sometimes thick blood has waste within it that creates toxic blood. Other times the blood is thick in the physical since which causes high blood pressure. When the thick blood is toxic prone it will over work the liver and damage the kidneys. If the blood becomes stagnant, **bad blood**, the tongue will be blue. Bad blood should be treated with sweet aromatic herbs such as sassafras or angelica. A tongue that is thick indicates thick blood that may be thinned from sweet fragrant herbs. If the tongue is thick and coated, the blood is turning bad.

If the blood settles in the legs it will create varicose veins, and dark spots around the ankles. This is called **low blood**. The skin will be dry and pale. The tongue will be dry. One may feel dizzy upon rising up. Confusion and memory loss may also occur. Use herbs that stimulate making the blood rise up such as elderberry and sassafras.

High blood is a condition where an excess of blood exists. The face and ears might be a light red. The skin will be warm to the touch. The tongue may be long darkened with a red end. One may be ill in the stomach, faint or have nose bleeds. A cooling fragrant herb should be considered like peppermint or angelica.

When one has a rapid heartbeat and a fever is present the blood has become **fast blood** and the fever indicates a problem. If the fast blood goes on for too long, the condition becomes sepsis. The infection must be addressed quickly. The tongue will be a dark red in this case. Use stimulating antiseptics like Virginia snake root.

When one has a chronic illness, they may eventually suffer from **slow blood**. Slow blood can delay recovery from a lingering illness by making the person feel slow and tired. Treat it similar to thick blood.

Cold blood is like a chill that will not go away. It makes the organs slow and they become coated with mucus. Use warming herbs with a bitter taste.

Nine

Color of Plants

The color of plants must be observed for they hold the secrets of the sun within them. All beings must partake of colorful foods to maintain health. Each color tells a wise potion maker what foods must be eaten to achieve wholeness.

Green is the color of life. It holds the very strength of the sun. Green plants give strength and energy. It also helps to build immunities and flush away impurities.

Yellow is the color of within. Yellow is a warm color and strengthens the linings around the organs in the upper body. It will increase the coating in the digestive tract.

Orange and Bright Red fruits and vegetables are warming. They are the colors of the setting sun. They help to control cancers and lesions and increases blood flow.

Dark fruits like **Blacks** or **Dark Reds** are cooling as they are of less light or not bright colored. These foods lessen susceptibility. They help blood move and reduce swelling. They relax muscles and reduce inflamed limbs.

Berries strengthen and protect the blood system. They help the heart and reduce pressure. **Cherries** help defeat the pain of gout.

Ten

Doses

Doses provided with nature must always be as small as possible. The magic in nature is very powerful and spans many areas. Potions that detoxify should be limited to the time it takes to perform their function. Potions that are used to change the spirit as well as the body should even be used less. Some of these potions may reside in the body for years. Infusions and decoctions are normally weak enough to consume a cup of potion. Many times the bitter taste is eased by the use of honey and the potion is consumed as a cup of tea.

Tinctures are much more concentrated and the use of one to three drops in a cup of water is common. Commercially processed tinctures have doses from ten to thirty drops per dose. Because of the potency of a tincture, they should not be given to children.

Children should never be given a potion by an apprentice potion maker. A child, being fresh in nature, has a purity built in and a master of potions or an experienced healer must be consulted before a potion is given.

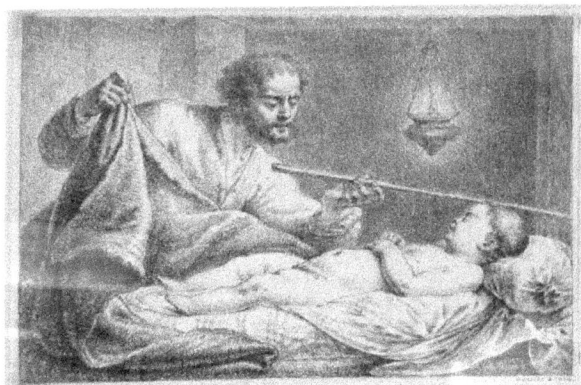

Common Herbs

While collecting material for potions, be sure you have selected the correct plants. Some plants are very similar in appearance to common herbs yet are deadly. The illustrations in this book are not intended for identification.

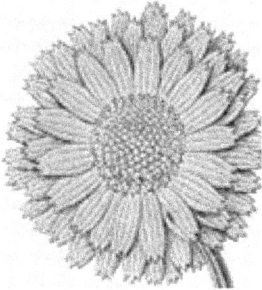

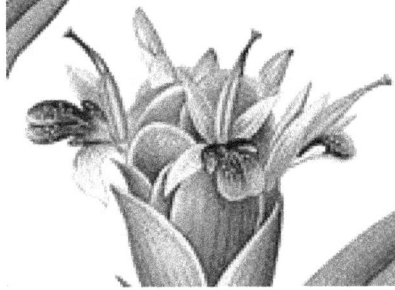

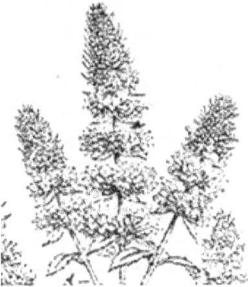

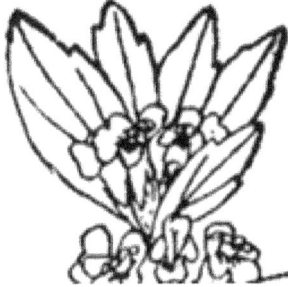

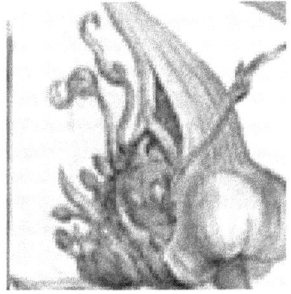

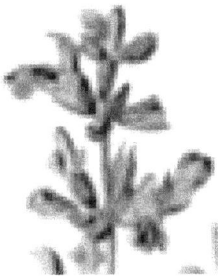

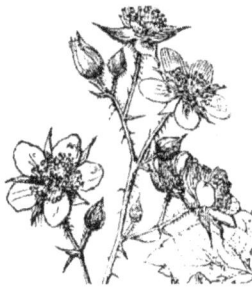

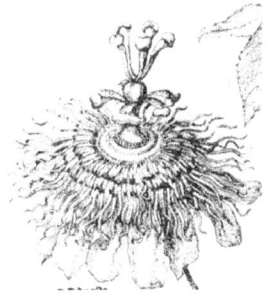

Calendula Officinalis (calendula)

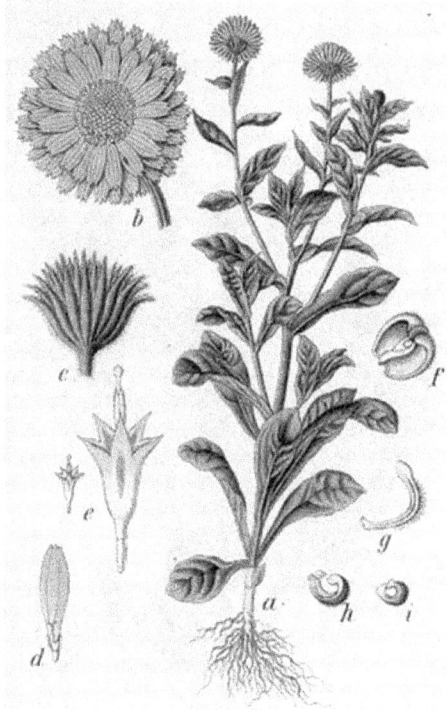

The pot marigold reduces swelling from insect bites, bruises and wounds and controls spasms in muscles. It is an astringent, which means it causes shrinkage of tissue to stop bleeding topically. It is beneficial for open wounds as it promotes growth of tissue. It helps to clear bile and toxins when taken internally. It removes pain of rashes, dry skin, earaches and ulcers.

All of this herb is edible and may be used internally or topically. Calendula may be used fresh or dried.

Taste – sweet, bitter salty, pungent – warm – astringent

Allium Sativum (garlic)

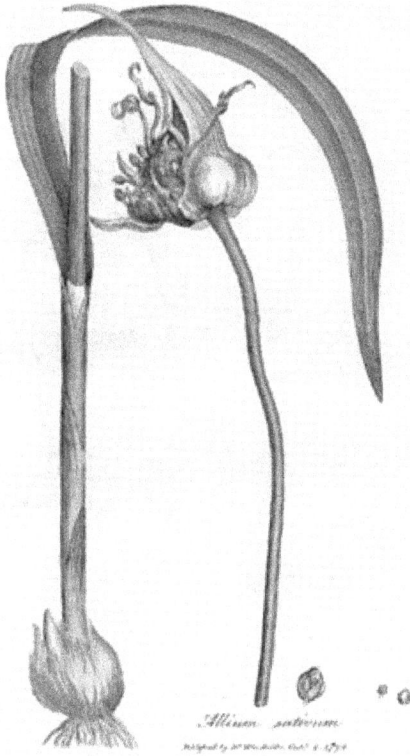

Allium sativum

Garlic will provide relief from bronchitis, chest congestion and help build immunities. It dispels cold and dampness.

The tuber is used internally and externally. An oil infusion rubbed on the soles of one's feet will relieve chest congestion. A clove swallowed daily will keep bronchitis at bay and build a strong immune system.

Taste – pungent, sweet, salty – warm, moist – stimulating

Zingiber Officinale (ginger)

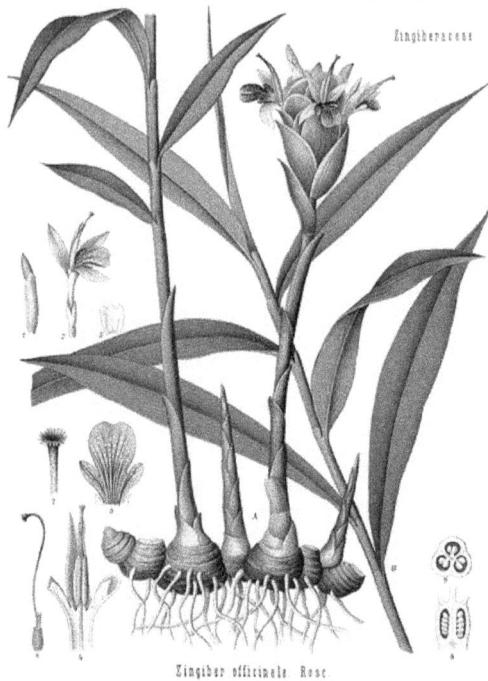

Zingiber officinale Rosc

Ginger eases nausea in light doses, settles the stomach in light doses, and helps with indigestion and gas. It will ease symptoms of colds when combined with lemon or honey and reduces sore throat pain in a honey infusion. Ginger expels mucus and increases circulation.

The tuber of this plant is used in primarily internal potions using dried and crushed materials. The root is very potent when fresh and may cause nausea if too much is eaten.

Taste – pungent, sweet – warm, moist – aromatic, stimulating

Salvia Officinalis (sage)

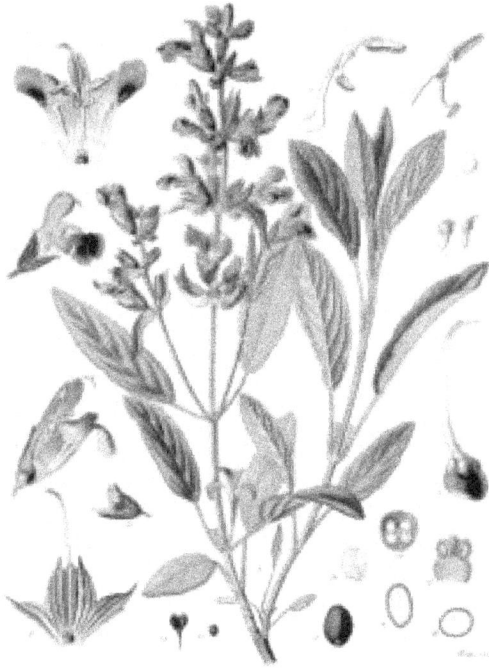

Sage is very commonly used in cold infusions made for topical applications. It has been the first herb placed into medicine bags to treat abrasions while on the trail along with other benefits. Internally it helps swollen glands, sore throat, fever and it thins the blood. Avoid prolonged use.

Sage has a long list of properties. It is an antibiotic, antifungal, astringent, antiviral, antispasmodic and anti-inflammatory. It is a natural insect repellant, even though bees are attracted to it. Sage honey is a natural aromatic.

Taste – pungent – warm – astringent

Thymus Vulgaris (thyme)

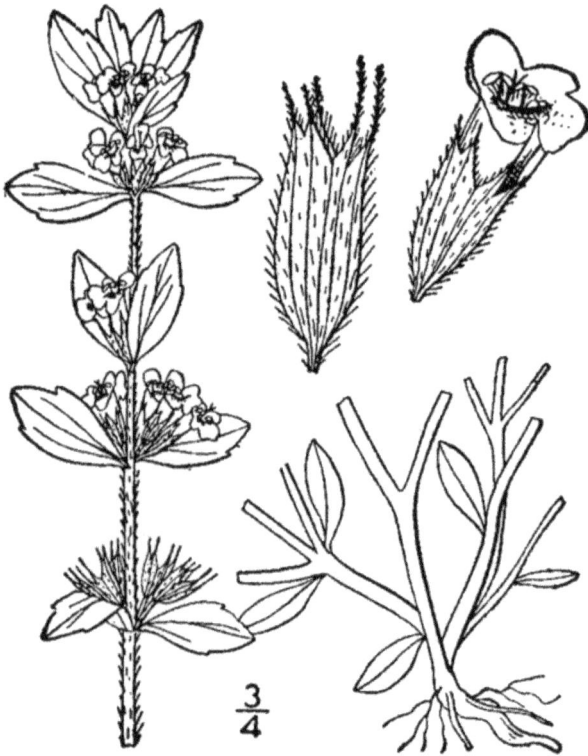

Thyme is drying and aromatic. Make a tea from the leaves for internal use for ailments of the stomach and digestive tract. Use to treat hook worms and other intestinal parasites. Use for bronchitis and respiratory infections by breathing in the steam of a thyme tincture. Cough medicine can be made with honey infusions.

Do not exceed two doses per day internally or one dose per day externally.

Taste – pungent – hot, dry – stimulating

Menthe Piperita (peppermint)

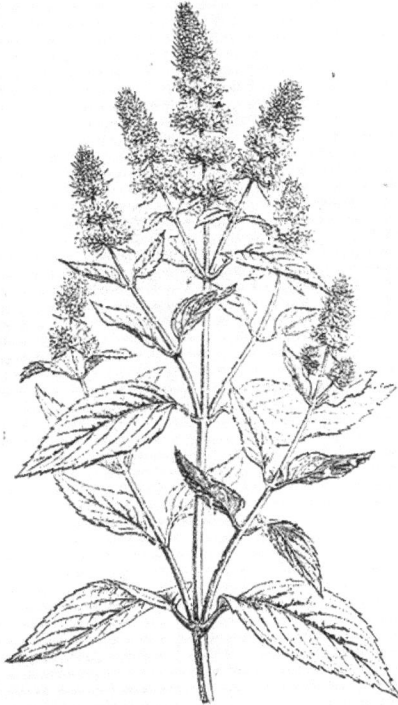

Menthe.

Peppermint has a long history of medicinal use where stomach ailments occur. A tea or tincture taken orally will relieve many aches of the stomach. It will help alleviate colic, and gas. It is a diuretic, anti-inflammatory, antispasmodic, antipruritic, mild decongestant, insect repellant and it is aromatic.

Note that spearmint is milder and would be more appropriate for infants.

Taste – pungent – warming and cooling – stimulating

Aloe Barbadensis (aloe vera)

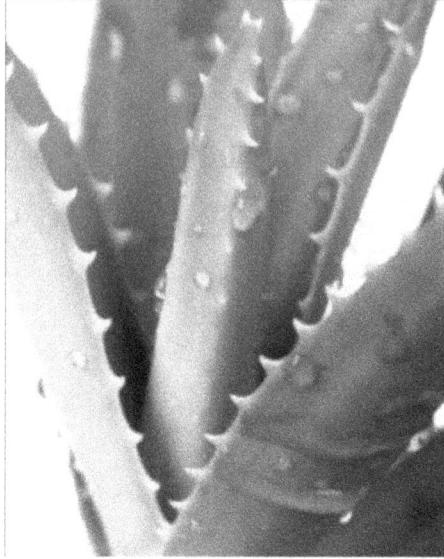

The cooling gel within the leaves of the Aloe Vera are antibacterial, anti-inflammatory, antifungal and aids in growth of tissue from 2nd and 3rd degree burns. It helps in healing of abrasions and heals gastric tumors. The gel mixed with water cools the intestinal lining and esophagus as well as the bowel.

Removing the gel within the leaves must be carefully executed. Within the outer skin lies a yellow latex material the plant uses as a defense mechanism. It is an irritant and also has laxative tendencies. Use small portions of the gel for internal use. Cut pieces about the size of a kernel of corn to the size of an average grape. Too much taken at one time will have the opposite effect when attempting to treat disorders of the digestive tract. The gel applied topically will aid in treating all contusions, abrasions, burns and sores, especially for diabetics.

Taste – sweet, salty, cool, and moist

Matricaria Discoidea (chamomile)

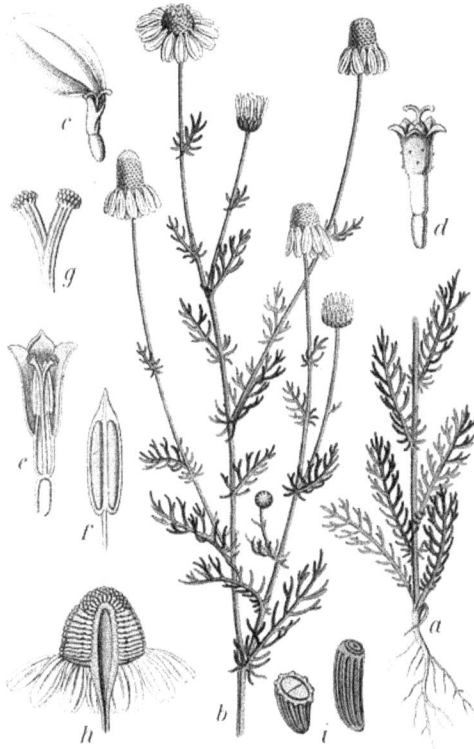

Chamomile is most commonly used to relax the body and mind when one is anxious or whiney. An infusion with small doses or aroma therapy may be used. Do not allow women with child to consume. It can trigger allergies related to ragweed and may also increase appetite.

This herb is an anti-inflammatory for mucus membranes and other tissue. It is an antispasmodic for the stomach.

Taste – sweet, pungent, bitter – cooling, drying

Sassafras Albidum, (sassafras)

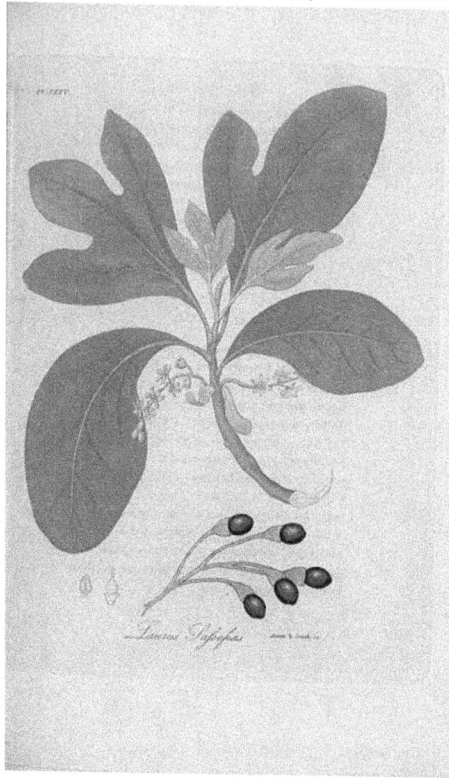

The root bark aids in digestion. Powdered root bark aids in healing bruises and swellings. It is a blood thinner and must be used with great care when taken internally for carcinogenic properties are said to be present.

A cup of sassafras tea made of the root bark thins the blood. Finely ground inner bark of the root used as a poultice on a bruise will prevent clotting of the blood.

Taste – sweet, spicy – cooling and warming – stimulating

Origanum Vulgare (oregano)

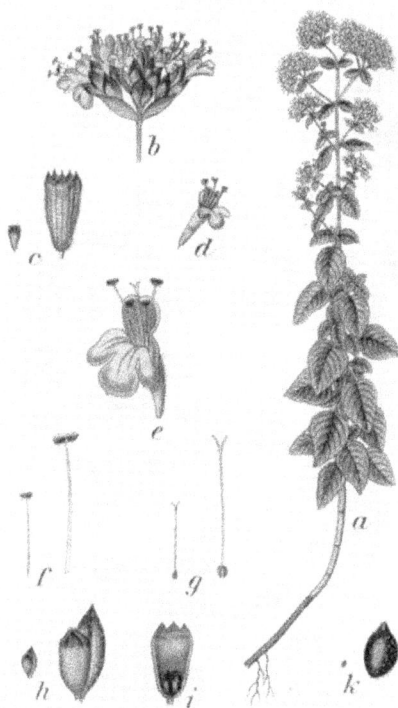

Oregano is cooling and moist. A decoction of the leaves of oregano may be taken internally for issues of the digestive tract such as indigestion, flatulence, bloating and menstrual cramps. The leaves can be used topically as a poultice for muscle pain, sore joints or itching. The oil of oregano will help in killing and removing lice.

Use the leaves and stems with blooms on them.

Taste – sweet, spicy – warming

Ambrosia Artemisifolia (ragweed)

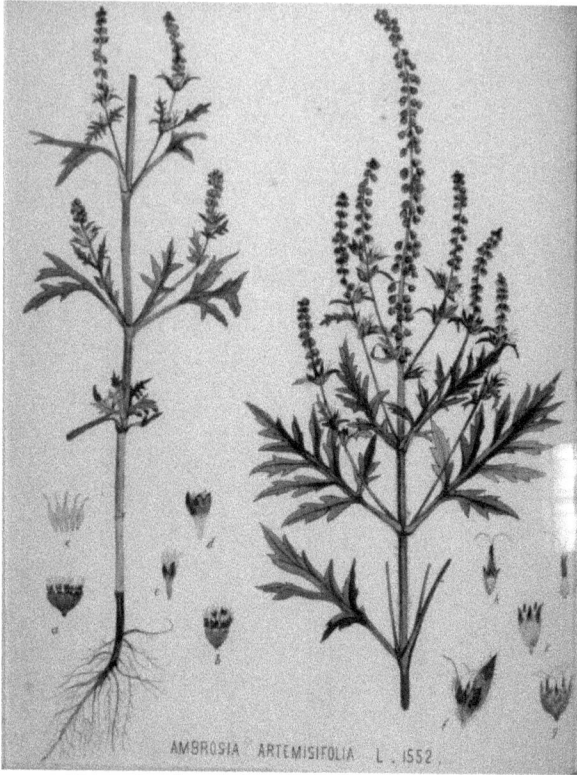

AMBROSIA ARTEMISIFOLIA L . 1552 .

Ragweed tincture is helpful when allergies begin when the pollen is in the air. The blooms, leaves and alcohol will need to be made the year before as it needs to sit for six weeks before it is ready for use. The plant is edible and the seeds are very digestible.

Taste bitter, pungent and astringent

Capsicum Annuum (cayenne pepper)

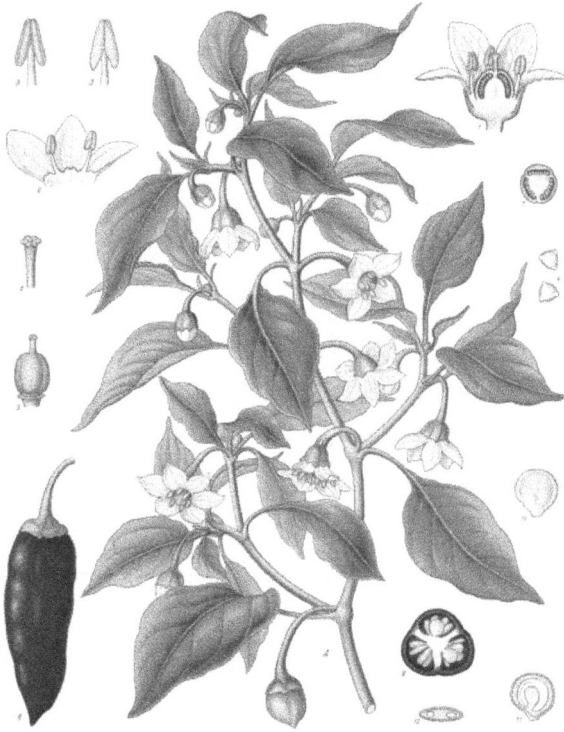

This herb tends to equalize blood pressure and improves blood circulation. Applying to a cut in powder form will stop bleeding quickly, even in deep cuts.

Also used for gas, stomach aches, cramping and constipation. A teaspoon of cayenne pepper in a cup of warm water is known to stop a heart attack. Cayenne is said to be the most powerful herb known today.

Taste – pungent hot

Rubus Villosus (blackberry)

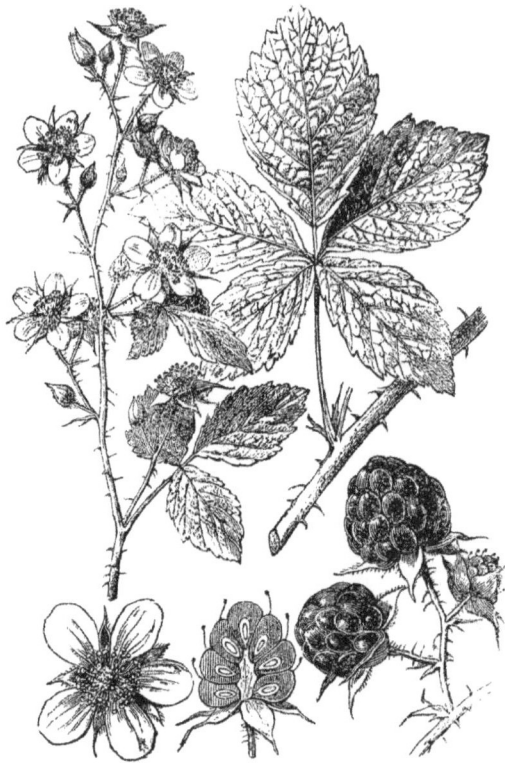

The leaf strengthens the stomach and intestines. Root bark in a decoction has the power to stop looseness in the bowels, help hemorrhoids, dysentery and other gastrointestinal disorders. A decoction with honey is good for a sore throat.

Blackberries are low in sugar and high in fiber making it very friendly to people with diabetes.

Taste – sweet, sour – cool, dry – astringent

37

Juglans Nigra (black walnut)

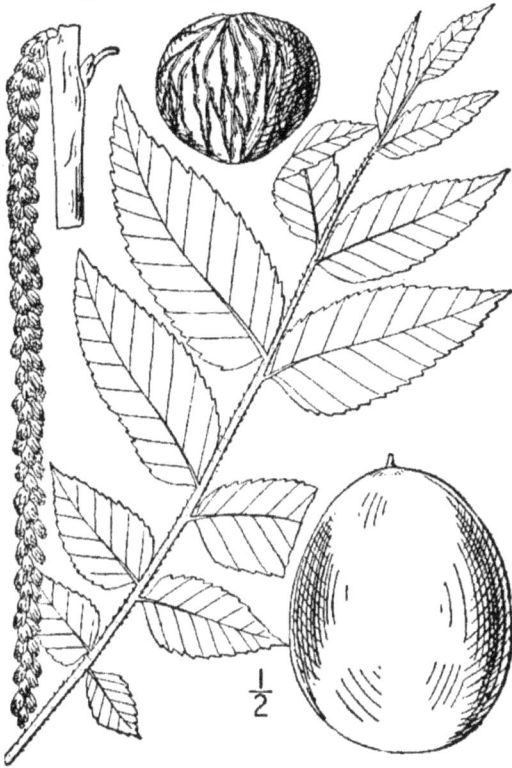

An infusion of the leaves or of the green hulls aid in the balance of the digestive tract. The hulls contain iodine and aids in the balance of the thyroid. The bark has stronger magic that affects the blood.

Leaves were used to drive away biting insects within bedding.

Taste – bitter, astringent

Passiflora Incarnate (passionflower)

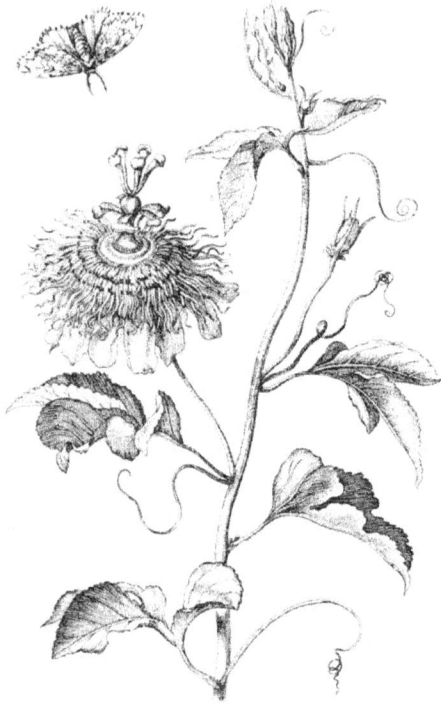

An infusion of the blooms will aid in relaxing the spirit within the mind by quieting the voices. Strong sedative qualities aid in nervousness, anxiety, gastrointestinal upset and seizures.

Passionflower infused honey is said to be the most gentle digestion aid.

Taste – sweet, sour

Juniperus Communis (juniper)

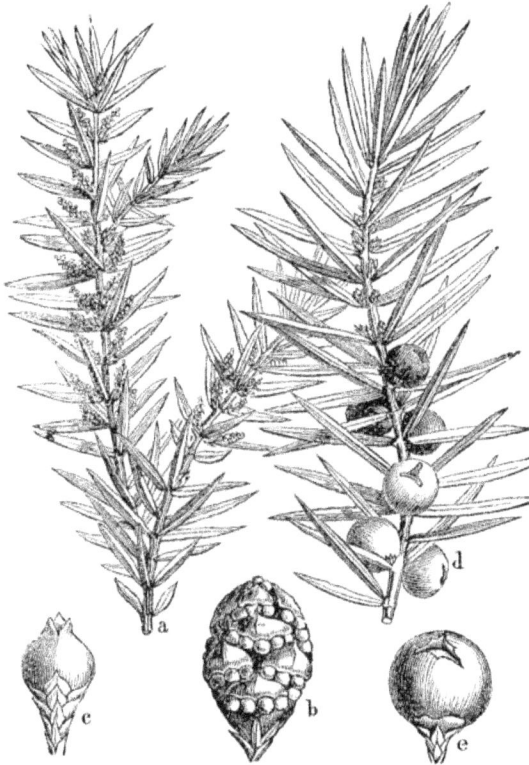

Juniper berries are used as a diuretic. They also are used in chronic renal congestion with back ache. They are also good in stopping water retention, especially in the lower body.

The antiseptic qualities and volatile oils aid in treatment of insect bites.

Taste – bitter, acrid, pungent, sweet – warm, dry – oily aromatic, antiseptic

Helianthus Annuus (sunflower)

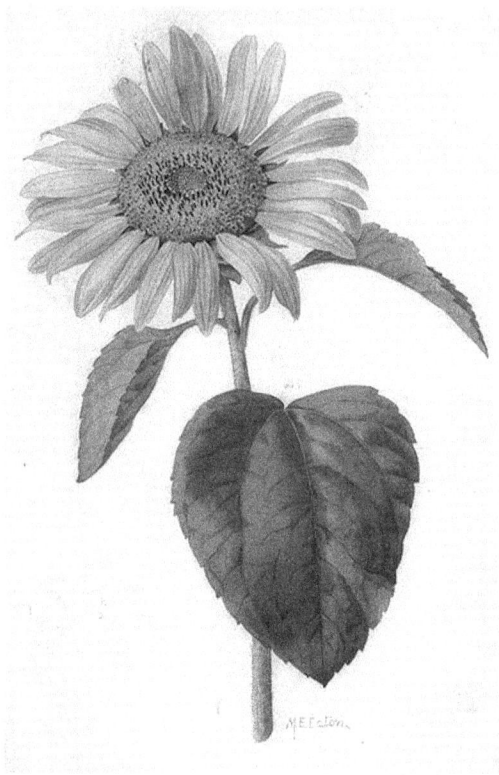

The seeds and oil from the seeds is a strong detoxifier for the upper respiratory system. Use for a persistent dry cough and early tuberculosis. It is moistening, so do not use with a cough caused by drainage of phlegm.

Taste – sweet

Notes:

Notes:

Notes:

www.ingramcontent.com/pod-product-compliance
Lightning Source LLC
Chambersburg PA
CBHW020953030426
42339CB00004B/74